ABOUT THE AUTHOR

Student and artist Ruby Warner shares her own
mental health journey through honest and
heart-warming illustrations on Instagram,
in the hope that what helped her may help others.

Ruby regularly works with mental health and suicide
prevention charity Beder, and collaborates with
Selfcareisforeveryone to create designs for apparel.

Find Ruby at...

Instagram @worrywellbeing

Etsy @worrywellbeing

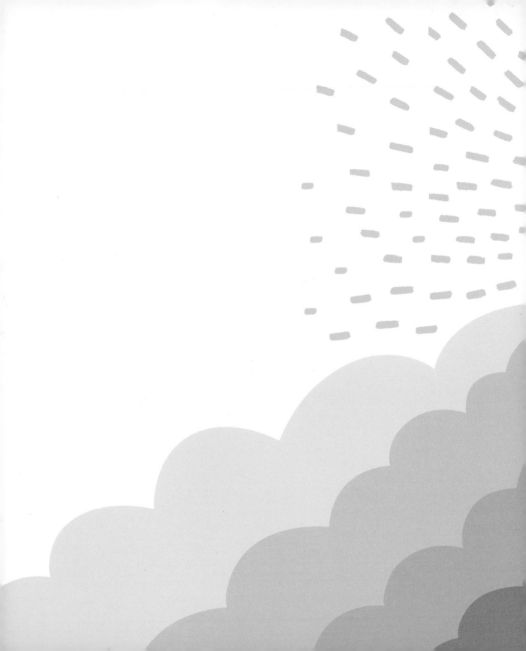

LITTLE
MOMENTS
OF LIGHT

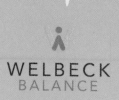

WELBECK
BALANCE

LITTLE
MOMENTS
OF LIGHT

Finding glimmers of hope in the darkness
and embracing everything in between

RUBY WARNER

Foreword by Suzy Reading

Published in 2022 by Welbeck Balance
An imprint of Welbeck Trigger Ltd
Part of Welbeck Publishing Group
Based in London and Sydney
www.welbeckpublishing.com

A CIP catalogue record for this book is available from the British Library.

ISBN
Trade Paperback – 978-1-80129-155-2
Hardback – 978-1-80129-257-3

Typeset by Jenny Semple Design
Printed in Dongguan, China by RR Donnelley

10 9 8 7 6 5 4 3 2 1

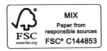

MIX
Paper from
responsible sources
FSC® C144853

Note/Disclaimer

For all those searching for hope.

Foreword

It is a true joy to welcome you to *Little Moments of Light*. Whether you are brand new to Ruby's work or perhaps, like me, you've been avidly following @worrywellbeing on Instagram, I am delighted that this book brings you Ruby's compassionate wisdom – a beautiful book to cherish yourself and one to gift widely, because we all need a little tenderness.

The kind companionship you'll find in this book makes all the difference. Welcome to walking the path together within these pages, enjoying the calm reassurance from a voice who knows.

As a chartered psychologist, self-care advocate and author myself, I deeply admire Ruby's work; her illustrations skillfully convey a thousand words.

In addition to soothing and uplifting art, you will find meaningful prompts, powerful mantras, loving reminders and the essential skills for managing difficult emotions, with Ruby guiding you step by step.

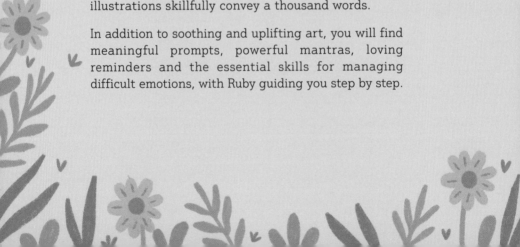

I love that Ruby doesn't shy away from telling it like it is, but at the same time plants seeds of hope, instils belief that things can get better and empowers with the practical tools to make purposeful change.

Read it cover to cover, or open any page at random, and you'll find the perfect inspiration, meeting you wherever you are at.

Even in the heaviest of times, I believe Ruby will reach you – normalizing and validating your feelings, helping you feel understood and less alone.

Most importantly, throughout the pages of this honest and heartwarming book you'll be reminded of your deep abiding self-worth. Let the comfort begin.

Suzy Reading

Psychologist and author of *The Self Care Revolution*
@suzyreading

Contents

you are going to get
through this and find a
brighter tomorrow

Introduction

I want to start by telling you what this book is not. This book is not going to tell you How to be Happy, or the 10 Steps to a Perfect Life, or what you need to do to Combat Stress. As someone who has experienced mental health struggles, I know how patronizing and unhelpful those words can be. I know how frustrating it is to be told that your anxiety can be cured if you "learn to breathe properly" or your depression will vanish if you just "think positively".

What I want this book to do is meet you where you are, wherever that may be, and remind you that everything will be OK. That it is OK to feel things, even the overwhelming and confusing things. And that even when you're in a dark place, things can and will get better.

This book is for you, wherever you are with your mental health. Perhaps you're having a "down day" and need some words of comfort and reassurance. Perhaps you've felt yourself struggling for a while and really want to pull yourself back into a brighter place. Or perhaps you're stuck in a really dark place, with no end in sight and feeling at rock bottom. I've been in all of those places, and I'm still working on it.

My hope is that this little book will make you feel a tiny bit brighter.

Finding Hope

there is
always hope,
even when you
don't feel so
hopeful

When we are struggling, feeling hopeful can seem impossible. I remember longing to be happy, but not believing this would ever be a possibility. I felt stuck, doubtful that things would ever change or get better.

It can take a bit of searching, but there is hope to be found even in the darkest of places.

Even on the days when it is a struggle to get out of bed, we can still appreciate the sun flooding through the window or the comfort of a soft blanket. When everything feels heavy and overwhelming, we can try to focus on the little ways we can help ourselves feel a little better, a little lighter.

On the difficult days, let yourself feel the sadness, the anxiety, the frustration. Accept that things are tough right now, but know that it won't feel like this forever. Things will get better. There is always hope. Even when you don't feel so hopeful.

Hope is...

- Trusting that things can and will get better
- Acknowledging the bad things, but looking for the little moments of good
- Choosing to get up each morning and carry on, even when things feel difficult

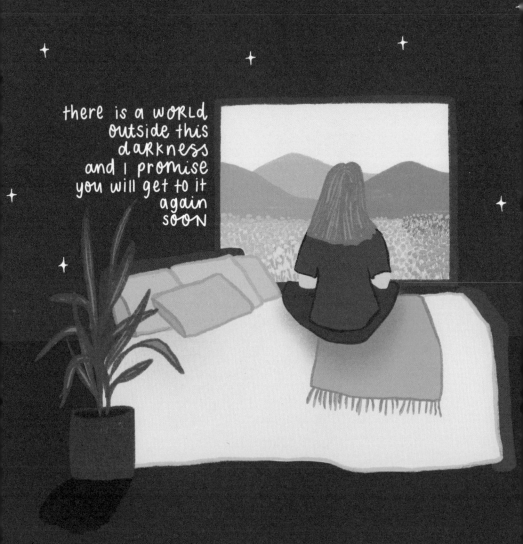

there is a WORLD
outside this
darkness
and I promise
you will get to it
again
soon

6

SITTING IN THE DARKNESS

I remember sitting in the darkness that is depression. It is like looking at the world around you through a glass window. You can see other people laughing and enjoying themselves, you can see what happiness looks like, you can see the life you desperately want. But you cannot get to it.

I remember this feeling so vividly: being on the other side of the glass, able to see happiness but unable to reach it. I wanted to go out, see friends, walk my dog, study, make art, enjoy my life. But my body felt so heavy with the weight of sadness. The colourful view of the world outside felt distant as I sat in bed, the dark shadow of depression towering over me. I felt trapped and lonely. I couldn't see a way out.

I want you to know that you can – and will – escape the darkness.

Recovery from depression is hard, but it is absolutely possible. It doesn't happen overnight. There's no switch that flicks and one day you're happy again. There's no simple solution. But with time, patience and support, things can – and do – get better.

Keep looking out of the window. The happiness you want and deserve is closer than it may feel.

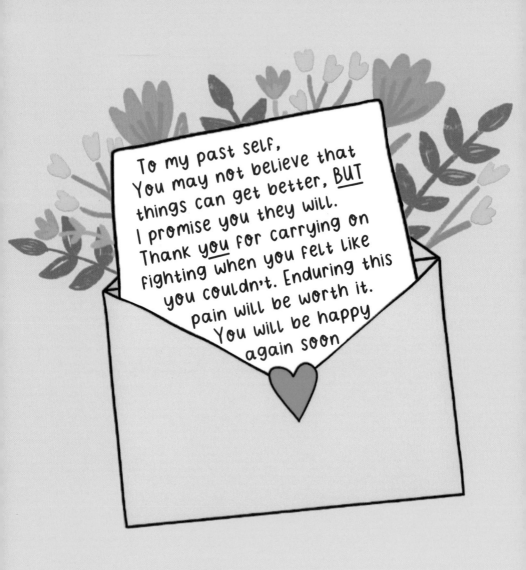

To my past self,
You may not believe that things can get better, <u>BUT</u> I promise you they will.
Thank y<u>ou</u> for carrying on fighting when you felt like you couldn't. Enduring this pain will be worth it.
You will be happy again soon

A NOTE TO MY PAST SELF...

If I could say anything to my past self, I'd want to say that it does get better. I'd want to thank my past self for carrying on, even when she felt like she couldn't. And I'd like her to know that carrying on, despite the difficult times, will be worth it.

So, this is your reminder to thank yourself for carrying on through the difficult times too. It's a brave thing, to keep going even when it feels like the hardest thing to do.

> Keep going. There is still so much more to experience. It's worth holding on for.

In this letter to my past self, I am talking directly to anyone who is struggling right now. Things get better. One day you too will be able to look back on everything you have overcome and thank yourself for carrying on.

Reasons to keep going...

★ There are so many places you haven't visited yet

★ There are so many kind people you haven't met yet

★ There are so many beautiful things you haven't seen yet

THE HOPE IN THE LITTLE THINGS

When I was struggling, I found it difficult to be hopeful. I found it impossible to see any positives at all. Seeing the good is not easy when you're in the depths of depression and anxiety.

Something that helped me was taking a few minutes at the end of each day to acknowledge any positive moments. I started keeping a little journal and I would write down something good that had happened that day, something I was grateful for, or just something small that made me smile.

Doing this helped me to start focusing on the good. I realized that even when I'd had a bad day, there were still happy moments within it. For example, one day when I was working as a waitress and feeling incredibly overwhelmed, I noticed a customer had left a note on their table before leaving. "Everything will be OK", it read. That tiny piece of paper made my day. When I got home, I stuck it into my journal as a reminder that there are good things and kind people amongst our everyday stress.

Whenever I feel down, I look back through this journal at all of these little moments of joy and it gives me a sense of hope. (If journaling isn't your thing, you could fill up a jar with little notes of these happy moments.) It's not going to solve all your problems – it's not supposed to. But appreciating tiny moments of joy can help make each day a little better.

GRATITUDE PROMPTS

a person you are grateful for

a lesson you are grateful for

a place you are grateful for

a song or book or movie you are grateful for

a memory you are grateful for

something about yourself you are grateful for

little moments

watching your favourite film

getting into a freshly made bed

singing along to your favourite songs

creating something you are proud of

getting lost in a good book

cuddling your pet

watching a beautiful sunset

listening to the sound of rain on your window

# of happiness

eating your favourite meal

laughing with friends

finding a few song you love

hugging someone you love

wearing an outfit that makes you feel good

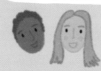

breathing in fresh air in nature

receiving a compliment

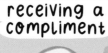

enjoying a hot cup of tea

you look lovely!

Finding Acceptance

Radical acceptance

♥ what can I do in this moment to help myself feel a little better?

♥ how can I make this situation more bearable?

♥ what words of comfort can I give myself right now?

There are a few different types of acceptance when it comes to your mental health: accepting emotions, accepting yourself, and accepting what you cannot control.

Acceptance is not always an easy process. Some things are incredibly difficult to accept, and that is OK.

Practising something called "radical acceptance" has very much helped me during difficult times.

Radical acceptance is when you accept that you cannot fight against reality. Instead, you focus on what you can do in this moment to make it more bearable.

This really resonates with me because sometimes all you can do is sit with the feelings and just do whatever you can to help yourself feel a little better. You can't stop it raining, but you can put your coat on and wrap up warm. It doesn't get rid of the bad weather; it does make things feel easier.

Acceptance looks like...

- Letting go of the things you can't control
- Sitting with uncomfortable emotions
- Allowing yourself to fail and make mistakes
- Appreciating your body for everything it does, regardless of how it looks
- Admitting you need help

i'm learning
to BE comfortable
Sitting with the
uncomfortable
emotions

ALLOW YOURSELF TO FEEL

I often get asked, "How do I stop feeling so anxious?", "What can I do to feel happy?", or "How do I get rid of this feeling?" It makes sense – we feel bad, and we don't want to feel bad, so we try to get rid of that feeling. We prevent ourselves from feeling anything uncomfortable or difficult.

Some people do this through avoiding situations that make them anxious; others might turn to unhealthy coping strategies to numb feelings of depression, or keep constantly busy to ensure that they are never alone with their thoughts. Whilst avoidance is a natural response to difficult emotions, giving ourselves space to feel them is so important.

We often resist and suppress our emotions, letting them build up until they are overwhelming and difficult to manage. This may come from the pressure we put on ourselves to be happy and positive all of the time – but this is incredibly unrealistic. Some days are hard and we feel sad or anxious, and that is OK.

Some emotions are very uncomfortable and difficult to accept, but it is important to remember that emotions cannot hurt you. As awful as it can feel to sit with the emotions, you can do it and the feeling will pass.

THIS FEELING WILL PASS

SITTING WITH DIFFICULT EMOTIONS

When difficult feelings arise, it is important to take a few moments to fully process and accept these emotions instead of ignoring them, squashing them down or trying to get rid of them. Below is a useful technique that you can use when experiencing overwhelming or challenging emotions.

The STOPP technique

1. **Stop.** Give yourself a moment to pause.

2. **Take a breath.** Give yourself a minute or so to breathe deeply and focus your full attention on your breath.

3. **Observe.** Notice how your body feels, recognize the thoughts you are experiencing and try to identify the emotions you are feeling.

4. **Put things in perspective.** Try to look at the bigger picture and think about whether you can look at the situation in a different way.

5. **Practise what works and proceed mindfully.** Choose an activity that helps you feel calm.

Letting yourself feel your emotions does not mean you are wallowing in them or feeling sorry for yourself. You are acknowledging how you feel and using healthy coping tools as best you can.

it's OK...

to say no

to take breaks

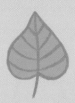

to put your mental
health first

to fail at
something

to have bad days

to feel angry
and upset

EMBRACING YOUR IMPERFECTIONS

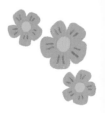

People often talk about the importance of self-love, but self-acceptance is a step that's often missed out. Before we can love ourselves, we have to accept ourselves. It can be a struggle to embrace all parts of yourself, even the parts you don't like, but it is possible to learn to accept your imperfections. There can often be barriers in the way of self-acceptance and so it is important to acknowledge these things in order to overcome them.

Things that might be in the way of self-acceptance...

- Expecting yourself to be perfect
- Comparing yourself to others
- Other people's comments/judgements
- Negative self-talk

Perfectionism often stands in the way of self-acceptance and this is something I have always struggled with. When you have impossibly high expectations of yourself, it can feel like nothing you do will ever be good enough. Learning to be comfortable with your imperfections is a very difficult thing to do, but we have to embrace these things in order to accept ourselves.

CHALLENGING NEGATIVE THOUGHTS

Is this thought completely true?

What would I tell a friend in this situation?

Am I blaming myself for something that is not my fault?

Am I jumping to conclusions?

Am I under-estimating my ability to cope?

How can I look at this situation differently?

SPEAKING KINDLY TO YOURSELF

Working toward self-acceptance often involves challenging negative thoughts and beliefs about yourself. When a negative thought arises, try thinking about how you would speak to a friend or a loved one and adopt this compassionate tone when speaking to yourself. You wouldn't tell a friend how ugly they looked or what a burden they have become. You wouldn't point out their imperfections. You don't deserve to be spoken to unkindly, so notice the way you speak to yourself.

Give yourself the same love, support and encouragement as you would give a friend. I know it's much easier said than done but being the voice you need to hear is so powerful.

Giving yourself words of comfort when you need them and learning to be gentle with yourself can be so valuable.

Practising positive self-talk on a daily basis can help us work toward self-acceptance. Start by catching yourself in moments of negative self-talk and replacing these thoughts with kinder ones. Or stick positive reminders around your house, maybe on your bathroom mirror or somewhere you frequently pass, to remind you to try positive self-talk. Repeating positive affirmations for self-acceptance (even if you don't believe them) can, in the long term, reframe some of the critical thoughts.

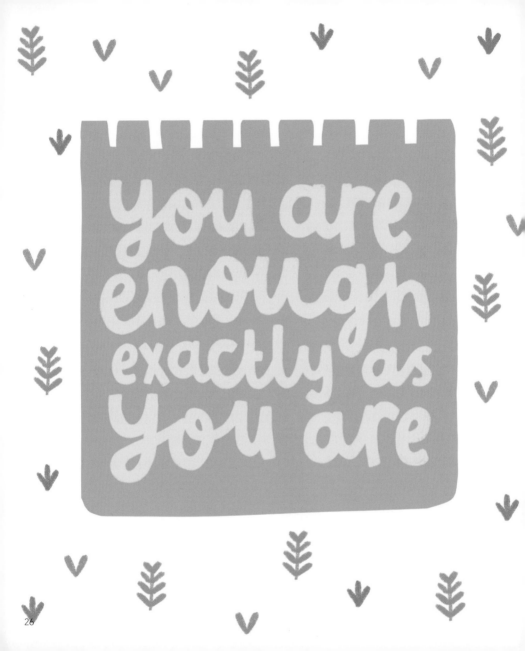

WAYS TO PRACTISE SELF-ACCEPTANCE

repeat positive affirmations about yourself every day

treat yourself with respect and kindness

try as best you can to stop comparing yourself to other people

write a list of things you like about yourself e.g., I always try to help others, I am hard working, I am creative

embrace your imperfections

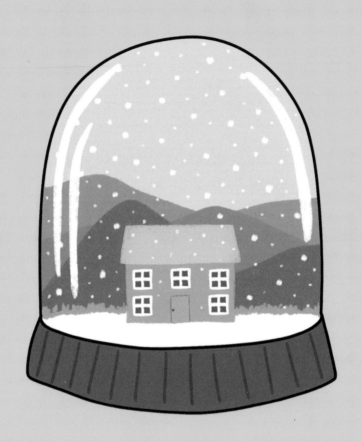

focus on the things you can control

ACCEPTING WHAT YOU CAN'T CONTROL

For me, a big part of acceptance is letting go of the things that I have no control over. As someone with anxiety, I struggle to accept that not everything is in my control. But letting go can be freeing.

I used to worry so much about other people's opinions and judgements. I would avoid so many things, I was always quiet in social situations – all out of a fear of being judged. But I've realized that people will have opinions whatever you do.

You will never please everyone, so you might as well focus on what makes you happy.

I used to try to fix people and solve their problems. I felt like it was my responsibility to make people feel better. But again, I've realized that other people's happiness is not solely my responsibility. You can support people, listen to them, be there for them through their difficult times. But it is not your job to make everything better.

You cannot stop bad things from happening in the world, you cannot prevent people from getting hurt, you cannot single-handedly stop the climate crisis, you cannot end all violence and inequality, you cannot be everything to everyone. But this does not mean you are powerless. You are powerful. With each little action, each word, each interaction, each smile, each act of kindness, you make the world a better place.

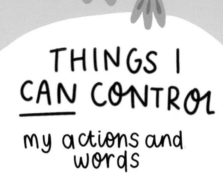

THINGS I
CAN CONTROL

my actions and
words

how I treat others

who I spend
time with

how I deal with
my emotions

the boundaries
I set

how I care for
my body

my beliefs and
opinions

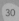

THINGS I CAN'T CONTROL

Other people's thoughts

time passing

that change is inevitable

Other people's actions

Other people's opinions

the past

Other people's decisions

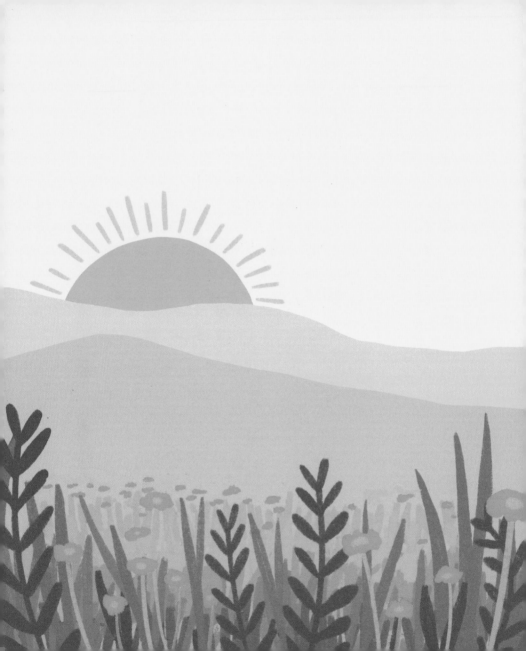

Finding Confidence

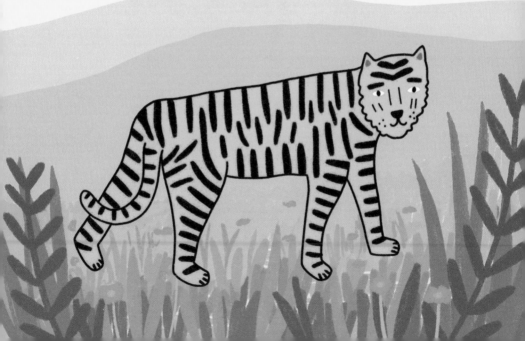

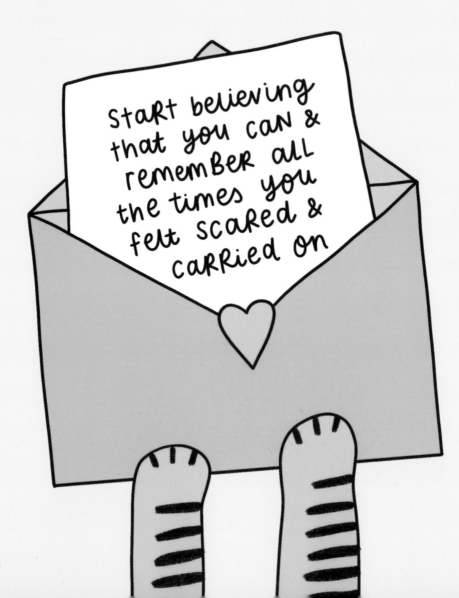

Learning to believe in yourself, have faith in your ideas and trust your own judgement is something that can take time.

There is a misconception that confidence means being loud, sociable, talkative, extraverted – and is accompanied by the need to be the centre of attention. But confidence is not an outward display of how sociable you are.

Being confident does not mean being the loudest person in the room. It means trusting yourself, pushing yourself and believing in yourself.

As someone who has lacked self-confidence in the past, I know how difficult it can be to overcome barriers when you lack self-belief. I struggled to voice my opinion, to put myself in new and scary situations, to step out of my comfort zone. But over the past few years, I have managed to do all of these things. So if you're feeling devoid of confidence, know that it is possible to believe in yourself again.

Confidence looks like...

- ★ Knowing your worth
- ★ Challenging yourself
- ★ Setting boundaries and saying "no"
- ★ Believing in yourself
- ★ Trusting that you can cope with difficult situations

CHALLENGING YOURSELF

One of the best ways to build confidence is to challenge yourself and to start facing the things that scare you. This might sound daunting, so it's important to remember to take things at your own pace.

Setting yourself little tasks each day is the best way of gradually facing your anxiety and building confidence, little by little. Each day, try to choose one small, manageable challenge to complete. That might be ordering a drink at a coffee shop, going for a walk by yourself or saying hello to someone at work. These may sound like small things, but if you repeat them frequently enough and make the challenges harder when you feel ready, exposure to the things that scare you can really help you overcome your fears.

When you are having low-confidence days, you can then look back on all of the brave steps you have taken and remind yourself how capable you are. I have a list of notes in my phone of everything I have done in the last year to challenge myself. Even small things like going to meet a friend when I wasn't feeling good about myself, or going somewhere new.

Each time you do something challenging, you are proving so much to yourself. You are proving that you are capable, that you can do hard things.

It takes a lot of courage to confront your fears. On many occasions, challenging myself has meant sitting with a great deal of anxiety. But being brave doesn't mean the thing you're doing doesn't scare you. Being brave is feeling that uncomfortable feeling and remembering that it will pass.

do things
that scare
you

Challenges for

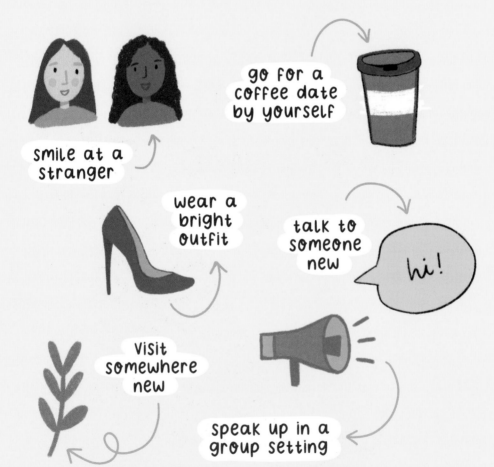

go for a coffee date by yourself

smile at a stranger

wear a bright outfit

talk to someone new

hi!

Visit somewhere new

speak up in a group setting

building confidence

take up a
new hobby

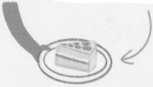

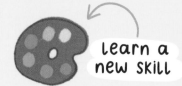

learn a
new skill

celebrate
your
successes

share your talents
with others

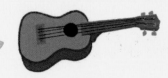

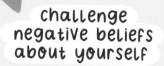

challenge
negative beliefs
about yourself

confront a
fear

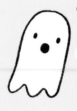

let yourself
feel the fear
but don't let
it stop you

AFFIRMATIONS FOR CONFIDENCE

I am capable

I can do this

I am confident

I am prepared

I am going to do a great job

I trust myself

I believe that I can

REMINDERS WHEN CHALLENGING YOURSELF

anxiety is uncomfortable but it cannot hurt you

you can cope with this feeling

you are capable of dealing with this

you can do this despite your anxiety

you will be so proud of yourself after

you can do this even though your head is telling you that you can't

you can...

♥ even when you feel like you can't

♥ even when you're scared

♥ even when you are doubting yourself

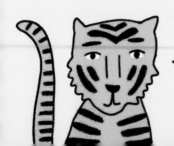

you got this

SAYING "NO" AND PROTECTING YOUR PEACE

An important part of having self-confidence is being able to say "No": being able to set boundaries and protect your peace. Practising setting boundaries and listening to what we need can help us to build confidence. If you are constantly letting people overstep your boundaries while ignoring your own needs, you are reinforcing the belief that you are not important. When we feel important, listened to and respected, we feel more confident. Stop shrinking yourself to make other people happy.

Maybe your friend keeps venting to you about their problems all of the time and it is making you feel drained and having a negative impact on your mood. Maybe someone at work keeps hounding you about a deadline when you've switched off for the weekend. Maybe you have said you can't attend a social event but people keep pressuring you to go, making you feel guilty for your decision.

You might feel like it's the right thing to do: keep everyone around you happy. But it's time to think about yourself, what you need and what will make you happy. You are allowed to say "No" and to set boundaries. Doing these things helps us grow in confidence.

Saying "No" to things that don't make you happy can be a liberating feeling. Listening to what you actually want, rather than automatically doing what you feel you should, can be very powerful.

SETTING BOUNDARIES

It is not my job to fix other people

I am allowed to take breaks

I don't need to explain or prove myself to anyone

It's OK to take time for myself

I am allowed to feel like this

It's OK to say no

I am allowed to prioritize myself

It's not my job to please everyone all the time

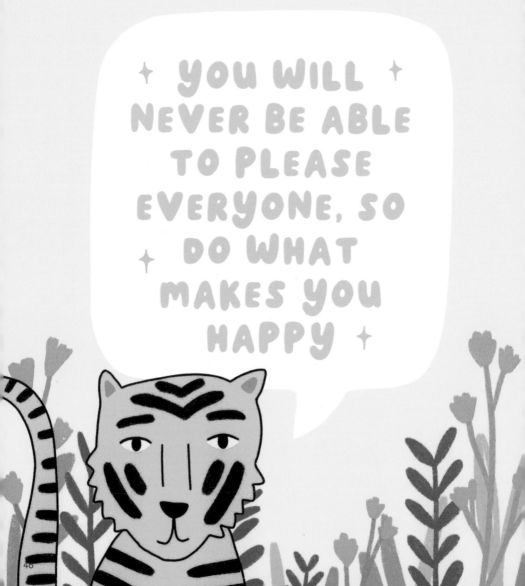

A note to people pleasers

 Stop changing yourself
for other people

 Stop saying "Yes" to things you are
not comfortable with or OK with

 Stop going out of your way for
people who make no effort

 Stop lowering your standards and
making excuses for people

 Stop ignoring your needs

 Stop apologizing for everything

Finding Calm

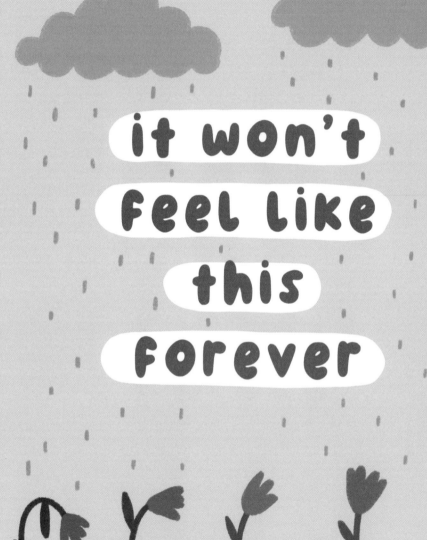

Anxiety is something I have carried with me for a very long time. I still carry it with me, but it is not as heavy as it used to be. Some days it feels bigger than others, towering over me and controlling everything I do. But mostly it is much more contained, taking up a lot less space in my life than it used to.

If you're thinking, "There's no way I will ever feel better", I have also felt like that. I know it's difficult to see how you will ever get out of the endless cycle of worry, how you will ever escape the awful physical symptoms, how you will ever be able to confront the things you are most afraid of. But I promise you it gets better.

There will be a time when you will get up in the morning without being overwhelmed by a feeling of dread. A time when you will be present in the moment and smile and laugh and really mean it. A time when you will be able to focus properly on a task. A time when you will fall asleep within minutes and not wake up with your heart pounding. A time when you will speak to new people.

There will be a time when you feel OK again.

Just as it isn't possible to be happy all the time, it's not possible to be calm all the time either – and accepting the ups and downs of my anxiety has been a big step toward getting better. Rather than trying to achieve a state of permanent zen (which is impossible to do), I try to focus on the little ways I can make myself a bit calmer and the little moments of peace I can find within the stress of everyday life.

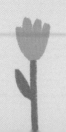
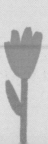
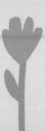

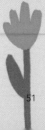

moments

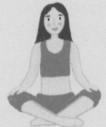

yoga/stretches

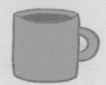

make a
warm drink

repeat
positive
affirmations

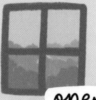

open a
window

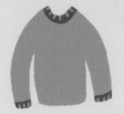

wear comfy
clothes

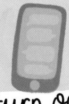

turn off
your phone

# of calm

take deep
breaths

notice your
surroundings
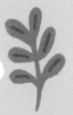

focus on
the present
moment

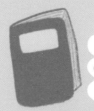
journal
about how
you feel

talk about
your worries

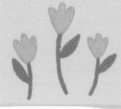
spend time
in nature

one step
at a time

REMINDERS FOR WHEN YOU FEEL ANXIOUS

you have coped with this feeling
before and can do it again

this feeling is uncomfortable
but it cannot hurt you

the physical symptoms will pass as
you calm down and breathe deeply

let yourself feel the anxiety

you are so brave for challenging yourself
and doing things despite being scared

Ride the waves

Anxiety, just like waves at sea, rises gradually, peaks, then falls.

When we begin to feel stressed, the wave begins to build momentum. It rises and rises until it reaches its peak. This is when we feel most anxious and panicky. After this point, the wave begins to fall and eventually fades away.

Instead of fighting against the waves as they come and go, I have learnt to sit with the discomfort and trust that the feeling will pass.

Learning our triggers and noticing the patterns in our anxiety can make it easier to anticipate when we might need to use our coping tools. For example, it can be helpful to begin to recognize situations and times of day you feel most anxious.

If you know you experience lots of anxiety in the mornings, then try making your morning routine as calming and gentle as possible, maybe scheduling time to practice yoga or meditation.

On the other hand, if your anxiety tends to increase more in the evenings, adjust your nighttime routine to include time to wind down or journal before bed.

Being curious, observant and getting to know your anxiety can help you better manage it.

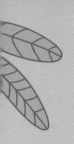

self

When we feel anxious, the best thing to do is to accept the feelings and sit with them – but we can still take steps to help ourselves feel a little better in the moment.

Doing things to help us feel calmer and more comfortable whilst we are experiencing such an uncomfortable emotion is very important.

Self-soothing is a powerful tool that can regulate anxiety. It involves engaging the senses to ground ourselves in the present moment.

Mindfulness is another tool that similarly involves focusing on the here and now and encourages observing emotions non-judgementally rather than labelling them as "good" or "bad".

Everyone is different, so what works for some people may not work for others, which is why it is good to try different things. Once you get to know what works for you personally, in anxious moments you can put these skills into practice.

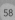

soothe

SOUND

- play relaxing music
- listen to a guided meditation
- open the window and notice what you can hear

TASTE

- have a calming herbal tea
- chew flavoured gum
- eat foods that help with stress e.g., dark chocolate, leafy greens, walnuts

TOUCH

- wear comfortable clothes
- have a warm bath
- lie under a soft blanket
- use a hot water bottle
- squeeze a stress ball
- stroke your pet

SMELL

- light a scented candle
- place a lavender bag underneath your pillow
- burn incense
- use a nice moisturizer
- use aromatherapy products

SIGHT

- turn on fairy lights
- set dim, warm lighting
- look at happy photos
- paint or draw
- observe your surroundings
- notice ten blue things around you

little moments

eat slowly

accept your emotions

objectively notice your thoughts

be curious

pay full attention

focus on the present

# of mindfulness

notice all five senses

practise using less judgement

do one thing at a time

listen carefully

be open minded

practise creativity

THE BREATH

Before I talk a little bit about the breath, I just want to reassure you that I'm not going to tell you to "Just breathe and your problems will be magically solved".

Breathing techniques are simply another skill we can call upon to help us during anxious moments. Here are a few of my favourite simple breathing patterns that I use (when I remember to).

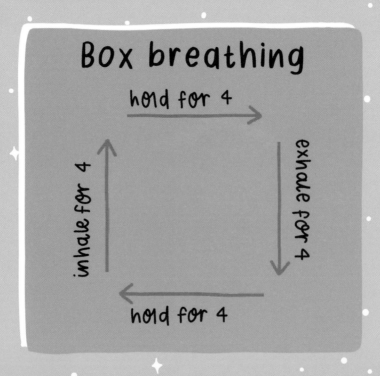

Gradual release breathing

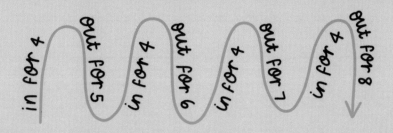

in for 4 · out for 5 · in for 4 · out for 6 · in for 7 · out for 7 · in for 4 · out for 8

4-7-8 breathing

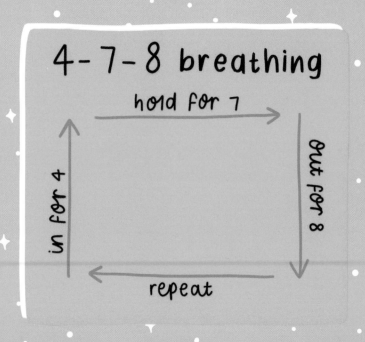

hold for 7

in for 4

out for 8

repeat

THE BODY

Our body carries anxiety in so many different ways. People often forget that mental health is very much physical too. It can cause headaches, heart palpitations, chest pains, loss of appetite, digestive issues, stomach pains, insomnia, fatigue, muscle tension, nausea and so much more. Experiencing these symptoms can be very scary, but if you are able to identify which symptoms you experience because of anxiety (and not because anything else is wrong), you'll find them much easier to cope with. Take the time to notice how anxiety shows up in your body.

Accept how your body feels. Listen to it. See it as your body's way of communicating that you feel stressed, and honour that feeling. Do whatever you can to make yourself more comfortable in that moment. Remember, it will pass.

Things that can help with the physical symptoms of anxiety...

* Yoga and stretching – to help muscle tension and body aches
* Exercise, such as running – proven to reduce anxiety and improve sleep
* Long deep breaths – lowers your heart rate and relaxes you
* Eating small, regular meals and plain food – helpful if you lose your appetite
* A regular sleep routine – to help with insomnia

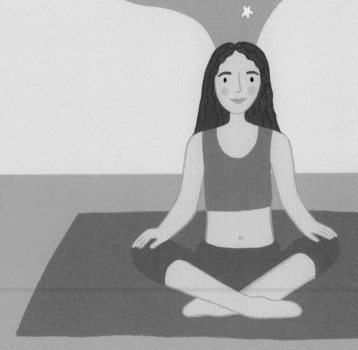

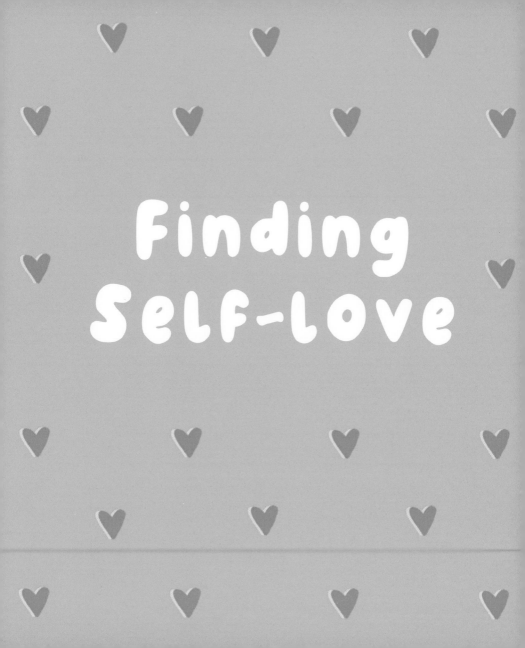

Finding Self-Love

When you think of self-love, your first thought might be face masks and bubble baths. And whilst these are valid forms of self-care, self-love is about much more than just how we take care of our physical bodies.

Self-love is about the way we view, treat and speak to ourselves.

This kind of self-love is something many people struggle with. When society is constantly telling us who we need to be, what we should look like and how to fit in, it's difficult to accept ourselves just as we are. When working toward self-love, we need to let go of these external expectations and focus on accepting and embracing who we are.

Reframing some self-love myths...

♥ **Self-love is not selfish.** Having a good relationship with ourselves can help improve our relationships with other people. When we take care of ourselves, we have more energy to take care of others too.

♥ **Loving yourself doesn't mean you think you are better than anyone else.** It means that you treat yourself with the same care and respect that you would treat others with.

♥ **Self-love can't be fully achieved through a good pamper session.** There is so much more to self-care than that. Self-love is about much more than just our physical bodies.

♥ **Self-care does not have to be time consuming.** It can be shown in something as small as mindfully making yourself a cup of tea, taking time before bed to wind down and read a book or going for a 20-minute walk. If you feel you haven't got time for self-care, it may be time to examine your priorities and commitments.

SELF LOVE IS NOT SELFISH

self-love

showing yourself
kindness even when you
feel bad about yourself

listening to yourself
and honouring your
needs

doing things your
future self will thank
you for

allowing yourself to
feel it all

looking after
yourself to prevent
burnout

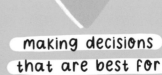

making decisions
that are best for
you

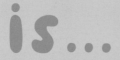

is...

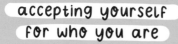

accepting yourself
for who you are

prioritizing the things
that are important to
you

taking a step back
when you feel
overwhelmed

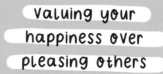

Valuing your
happiness over
pleasing others

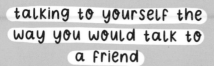

talking to yourself the
way you would talk to
a friend

letting go of the
things that don't
serve you

THE RELATIONSHIP YOU HAVE WITH YOURSELF IS THE MOST IMPORTANT RELATIONSHIP YOU WILL EVER HAVE

BUILDING A GOOD RELATIONSHIP WITH YOURSELF

Working toward self-love means improving the relationship you have with yourself.

Someone who has a good relationship with themselves knows their worth so will feel more confident standing up for themselves. They will find it easier to build healthy relationships and communicate with others.

How to improve your relationship with yourself...

⭐ Treat yourself the same way you would a loved one. If you wouldn't say it to a friend, don't say it to yourself.

⭐ Become comfortable in your own company. Spend time with yourself and get to know yourself. Connect with the parts of yourself you haven't discovered yet.

⭐ Be the person you need. Give yourself the words you need to hear. Be your own cheerleader, motivator, supporter. Be the one who comforts you through difficult moments.

⭐ Journal. It can be a great way of getting to know your inner dialogue, allowing you to reflect on your thoughts and emotions.

⭐ Let go of guilt. You are allowed to make mistakes and be imperfect. Being hard on yourself will only damage your relationship with yourself. Gift yourself patience and grace.

THINGS YOU SHOULDN'T FEEL GUILTY FOR...

- ⭐ Eating more when you are hungry
- ⭐ Not getting everything done
- ⭐ Taking breaks
- ⭐ Making mistakes
- ⭐ Asking for help
- ⭐ Being yourself
- ⭐ Saying no
- ⭐ Taking things at your own pace
- ⭐ Taking time for self care
- ⭐ Relapsing
- ⭐ Needing time alone

AFFIRMATIONS FOR SELF-LOVE

I am worthy of love

I accept and embrace myself for who I am

I am grateful for my body and all that it does for me

My worth is not defined by other people's opinions of me

I am enough

TAKING CARE OF YOURSELF

The little acts of self-care we practise on a regular basis almost act as the stepping stones to self-love. Each time we speak kindly to ourselves or take time to practise self-care, we remind ourselves that we deserve care and love.

Types of self-care...

- **Physical self-care** means how you look after your physical body, for example getting enough sleep, eating well, exercising.

- **Emotional self-care** is about dealing with your feelings in a healthy way, for example going to therapy, journaling, meditation.

- **Mental self-care** means engaging in activities that mentally stimulate you, for example cooking a new recipe, painting or drawing.

- **Social self-care** is about taking care of your relationships and connecting with others, for example meeting up with friends, spending quality time with your partner, calling a loved one.

- **Professional self-care** means looking after yourself in a work setting, for example setting boundaries, taking breaks, asking for help.

I often hear people say, "I truly don't have time for self-care", and I understand because I used to feel the same. But I then realized that self-care is as much about making the time, as it is about actually doing the act. Usually we don't make time for ourselves if we feel like we are not worthy of care and love in the first place. And the more regularly we practise self-care, the easier it becomes.

LITTLE ACTS OF
SELF-LOVE

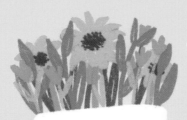

cook yourself
a nice meal

listen to your
favourite feel
good songs

spend some time
outdoors

think of three things
you like about yourself

buy yourself flowers

take some time to
reflect and set
some goals

let yourself
sleep in

write a list of positive
reminders and stick
them on your wall

go for a coffee date
by yourself

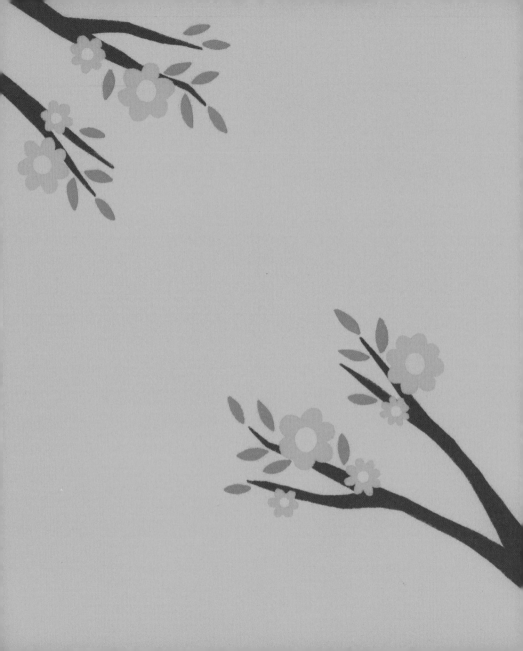

Finding Connection

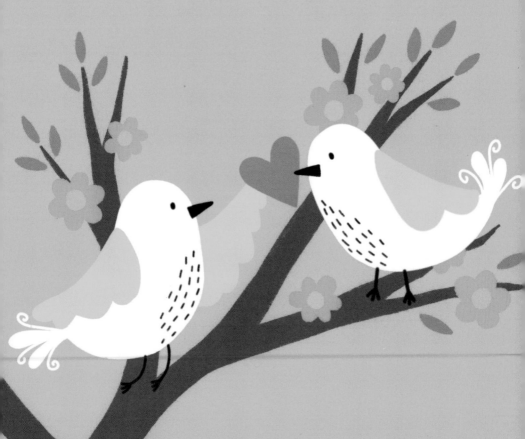

you are
not
alone

When I was really struggling with my mental health, I found it difficult to connect with people. I felt very angry with everyone and felt like no one understood. I found it difficult to communicate how I was feeling, especially as, at times, I didn't understand my emotions myself. I convinced myself that no one cared, which now I see was not the case at all. Lots of people loved and cared about me, but I couldn't feel it because I didn't love or care about myself.

> You have to believe that you deserve love and care, because you do.

It can be very isolating suffering with depression and anxiety. We tend to push people away. We might worry that we are a burden, feel like no one likes or accepts us, or just not have the energy to socialize.

I know it is challenging, but often in these times we actually need to do the opposite of what we feel like doing. I used to hide away at home, and ignore messages from friends. I closed myself off and withdrew. I did this because I felt sad and anxious, but all this did was make things worse. The more I closed myself off, the more disconnected and lonely I felt. It was a vicious cycle. And the only way of getting out of this cycle was to challenge myself. You have to do the hard thing sometimes. Talk to your friends. Go out. Join in as best you can. It's when you most want to hide away from people that you most need some kind of connection.

Relationships can be difficult to maintain when we're struggling...

you might have no energy to socialize

you might want to push people away

you might find it difficult to go out

you might worry that you will bring others down

you might worry that you are a burden

you might be more irritable than usual

... but it's important to remember...

⭐ you are not a burden

⭐ people still love and care about you, even when you don't love and care about yourself

⭐ pushing people away and isolating yourself will only make you feel worse

⭐ you deserve to have fun, to laugh, to enjoy spending time with people

YOU ARE WORTHY OF LOVE

Anxiety can make us doubt our self-worth and question our relationships. Maybe you feel like you are a burden to your friends, as if your partner is annoyed with you for no reason, or like no one wants you at social events. Maintaining relationships can be very tiring when you constantly overthink every interaction.

Low self-esteem can also cause us to believe that we don't deserve healthy, loving relationships. We often end up pushing the people who care about us away. But you do deserve support and you are not a burden. Of course, friends and family are not there to solve your problems, but they are there as a support network. It's OK to talk about what you are going through and to feel some relief from doing so.

You deserve to be listened to and supported.
You are not broken. You do not need to be "fixed".

There is so much more to you as a person than just what you are going through. I know what it is like to lose all sense of who you are when you are at your lowest. It feels like all you are is your illness – a big dark cloud that casts shadow over everything in your life.

You may not feel like it but all of the parts that make you special are still there. Your creativity, your kindness, your empathy, your sense of humour, your determination. You are still loveable. You just need some support and care right now.

ANXIETY IN RELATIONSHIPS

they're talking about me behind my back

I'm a burden

I'm a bad friend/partner

they're annoyed with me

I've done something to upset them

they're going to betray my trust

do they actually like me?

they don't want me here

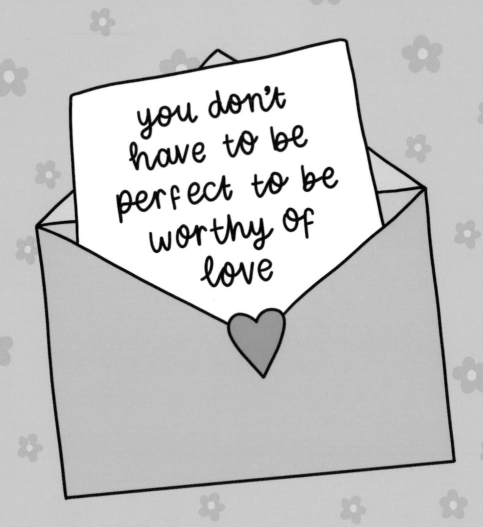

you deserve...

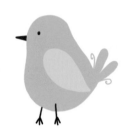

to be loved

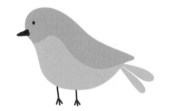

to be supported

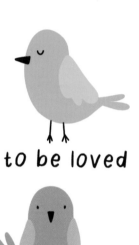

to be happy

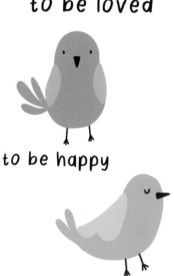

to be listened to

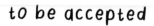

to be accepted

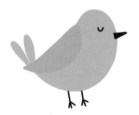

to be respected

COMMUNICATION FOR WHEN YOU'RE STRUGGLING TO TALK

Write a letter or send a text message explaining how you are feeling and what that person could do to support you

Think about the points you want to bring up and what you're going to say before you talk to them

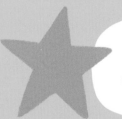

Let them know that you are finding it hard to talk right now

you haven't done anything wrong, I'm just finding it hard to talk right now...

SOCIALIZING WHEN YOU ARE STRUGGLING

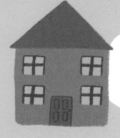

Ask if they can come and visit you at home if you feel anxious about going out

Meet in smaller groups if being with lots of people feels overwhelming

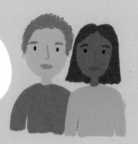

Talk to them about how you are feeling and explain that as much as you love spending time with them, it's a struggle for you to socialize right now

conversation

I'm really struggling with...

It would be helpful if you could...

I need help with...

I've been feeling...

I'm having a difficult time at the moment. I think I need some support with...

starters

I've been really worrying about...

I keep thinking about...

I feel really down and I don't know why...

I've been wanting to talk to you about...

I've been finding... more difficult than usual

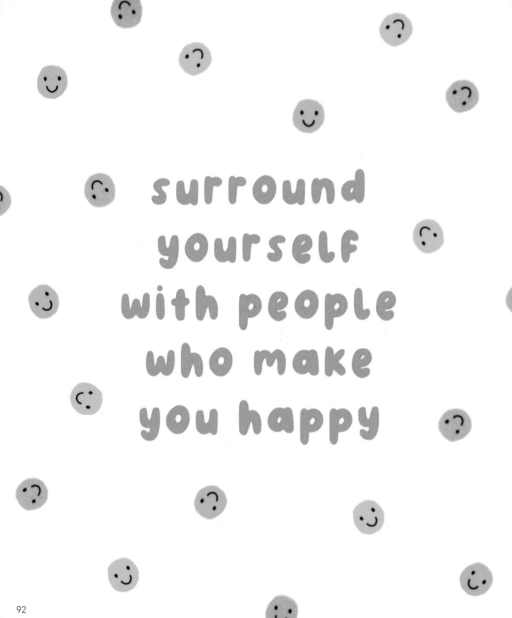

surround
yourself
with people
who make
you happy

FIND YOUR PEOPLE

The people in our lives have such a big impact on us, and this is why it's important to reflect on whether they are negatively or positively impacting us. Spending time with people who make little critical comments, or always find something to argue about, or never seem to be happy for you, can really affect your mood. It doesn't mean they are a bad person, but you are allowed to consider whether they are the healthiest person for you to spend time with.

Choose to be around people who uplift you, make you feel good and make you laugh — rather than people who drag you down.

Questions to ask yourself...

⭐ Do I feel happy after spending time with this person?

⭐ Does this person listen to me?

⭐ Does this person put the same amount of effort as I do into the relationship?

⭐ Do I enjoy being around this person?

If you are reading these questions thinking, "I have no one in my life like this", then please remember you are not alone. You might feel lonely right now, but you will find people who make you happy. There are so many people you haven't met yet and so many opportunities to develop new, positive relationships.

CONNECTING WITH NEW PEOPLE

volunteer at a charity shop, animal shelter or food bank

join a book club

join an online community

have lunch with a colleague at work

chat to other dog walkers on your walk

say yes to new experiences – you never know who you will meet

get to know friends of friends

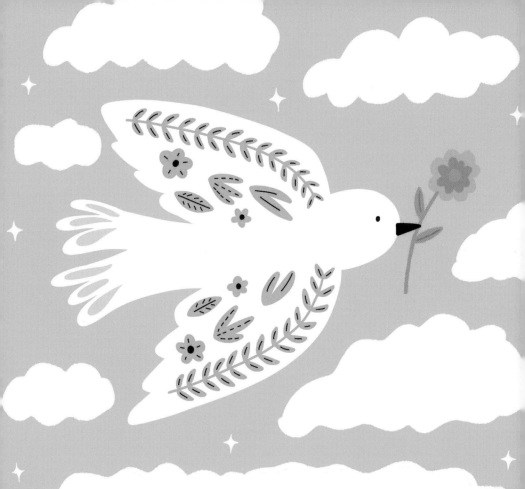

Connection is created through little acts of
kindness. It might just be a smile, a conversation,
a small gesture, but when we give others a
little light, we feel the warmth of it too.

little acts

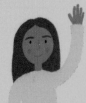

volunteer in
your
community

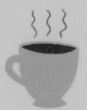

buy coffee
for a friend
or colleague

donate to
a food
bank

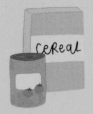

tell someone
you appreciate
them

give someone a
compliment

stick positive
notes on
mirrors

you
are
LOVED

# of kindness

 bake for someone

 carry around loose change to put in tip jars

TIPS

can I do anything to help?

give someone flowers

offer to help someone

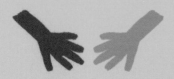 reach out to someone

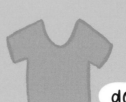 donate old clothes

FEARS WHEN REACHING OUT FOR HELP

no one will understand

people might think I'm being overdramatic

they might not believe me

what if they can't help me?

I might be judged

there are others who deserve help more than me

Finding help can be a daunting process. You might feel like you are not "bad enough" to get help or are worried that people will think you are being overdramatic. Maybe you are afraid of being judged, or are anxious that nothing will help you feel better. Maybe you don't want to worry people.

Whatever is holding you back, please know that reaching out for help is one of the bravest things you can do.

It might feel scary, but getting the support you need is the most important thing. This might look like setting up a doctor's appointment, finding a therapist, joining a support group or speaking to someone at work.

There are so many options when it comes to getting help that it can feel a little overwhelming! But having options means that if something doesn't work out, you can always try something else.

If you're struggling to know what to say, take a look back at "Conversation Starters" on pages 90–91 for some ideas of how to begin a conversation. It can also be useful to write a list of the points you want to bring up beforehand so that you don't miss anything important.

THINGS THAT CAN HELP

Getting outside in nature

Yoga

Meditation

Creating art

Journaling

Exercise

Herbal medicines

Listening to music

Talking to loved ones

Therapy

Mindfulness

Being around pets

Medication

whatever helps you is valid and important

NOTES ON THERAPY

It takes time to see the benefits of therapy

The more open and honest you are, the more you will gain

Therapy is hard work but it will be worth it in the long term

It might take time to find the right therapist for you

Going to therapy is nothing to be ashamed of

STARTING THERAPY

When you first start therapy it might feel a little strange opening up to someone you don't know, but therapy can be an amazing opportunity to learn and grow. You may not find the right therapist straight away and it can take some time to see the positive effects... but therapy can provide the tools you need to deal with difficult emotions and give you the space to talk about and process your experiences.

There can sometimes be a sense of shame or embarrassment that comes with going to therapy, but admitting that you need help and having the bravery to begin the journey to recovery in therapy is something to be proud rather than ashamed of.

Things I've Learned in therapy...

Showing yourself compassion is most important when you feel unworthy of love. It's in the moments we feel most unlovable, anxious, vulnerable, that we really need to show ourselves the same love we would show others.

Sometimes the thing that will help us feel better is the thing we least want to do in that moment. In these moments, you might have to make yourself go for a walk, practise self-care or reach out to someone, even when it's difficult.

Let yourself feel things. Listen to your emotions and what they are telling you and allow yourself to express how you feel.

With time and practise, you can face and overcome your fears. You are capable of more than you know and will one day do things you never believed you could.

REMINDERS WHEN REACHING OUT FOR HELP

you deserve support

everybody is unique and not everything will work for everyone

you are not weak for reaching out for help

you don't need to be at rock bottom or in crisis to seek help

there is no right way to recover

it can take a little while to find what works for you

Things that make me feel better:

♥ Everyone is different and unique, and so what works for one person may not work for another. There is no right answer when it comes to getting better; whatever helps you is valid and important.

♥ Personally, I have found multiple forms of therapy, including CBT, CAT and psychodynamic therapy, very helpful. Medication has also massively helped me manage my anxiety, depression and OCD.

♥ I love practising yoga regularly and find it helps ground me and reduce my physical and emotional symptoms of anxiety.

♥ I find getting out in the fresh air and taking my dog for a long walk very calming, as well as listening to music, watching comforting films and being with friends and family.

♥ What helps you feel better may not look the same as my list, but what matters is finding your combination of things that'll help you when you're experiencing difficulties.

Final Thoughts

I wanted to end with three things I hope you'll take away from this book.

1. It's OK to feel a lot

I want you to know that it's OK to feel things. It's OK to feel a lot.

We all have moments of anxiety, sadness, anger, frustration, stress and hopelessness. We also all have moments of laughter, happiness, peace, hopefulness, excitement, gratitude and optimism.

Allow yourself to feel all of these different emotions without guilt or shame.

2. You are not alone

I know it can feel lonely at times, but please remember that you are not on your own. There will always be people who care about you.

You matter. You are important. The world is a better place with you in it.

3. Things will get better

There was a point in my life when I was convinced things would never get better. The only future I saw for myself was one where I was sad and anxious and trapped by my mental illness.

You may not be able to see it right now, but things will get better. You have the strength to get through this. And I promise you that it will be worth carrying on.

Throughout this book, I have shared the things that help me and the things I have learned from my experience of mental health struggles.

I hope my words and art provide comfort, encouragement and most importantly, remind you that you are not alone in what you are going through.

I hope this book is something you can come back to when you are having a tough day; something you can pick up when you're feeling down or anxious.

Finally, I hope you have hope. Because even on the darkest of nights, there will always be little moments of light.

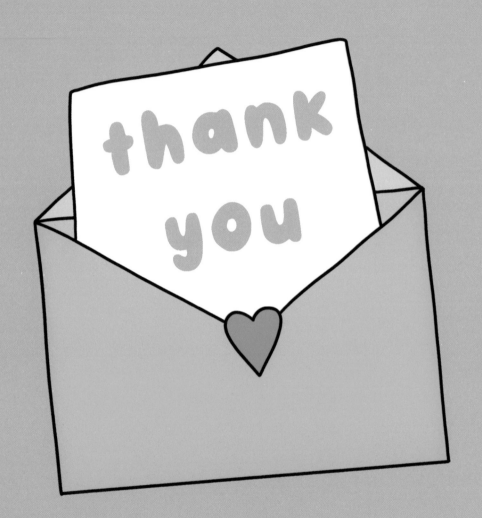

Acknowledgments

I would like to thank my parents and brother for being so supportive, not only throughout the process of creating this book, but also during the ups and downs I've been through over the past few years. Thank you, Mum, for being right by my side through it all, for listening to me, for being so patient with me even in my worst moments, and for being so caring and kind. Thank you, Dad, for always having so much belief in me, for sharing with me your love for reading and writing from such a young age, and for always reminding me how loved I am. Seamus, my little (but much bigger than me) brother, thank you for making me laugh and reminding me I'm loved, even if in strange ways. I'm so grateful to have such a loving family, both here and in Ireland. I can't forget to mention and thank my furry friend Arlo, for giving me endless cuddles and practically dragging me out of the house for walks.

Thank you to my beautiful friends, Liv G, Liv W, Ella, Mira, Ruby, Caitlin, Amy, Hannah and Carys, for being so supportive. You are all very special women who inspire me so much. Chloe, thank you for giving me laughter and light when I was at my lowest. Thank you, Jude, for being so supportive and caring. I'm very grateful to be surrounded by such positive and encouraging people.

Thank you, Tom, Vanessa and Dr Angeliki, for helping me get to the point I am at now and for playing such a big role in helping me get better. You helped me realize that I was capable of challenging myself, overcoming my anxiety, and being happy and confident again.

Thank you to my teachers for helping me gain so much confidence. Alex, thank you for pushing me to create art I was proud of. Lesley, thank you for opening up a whole world of social issues and empowering me to make a change in the world. Darren, thank you encouraging me to speak up and helping me realize my voice and words are valuable.

Thank you, Razzak, for welcoming me into the world of Beder. I feel very privileged to work with such a fantastic charity that does such valuable work in the memory of a very special person.

I would like to say a huge thank you to Welbeck for allowing me to bring this book to life, especially to Jo, Beth and Jenny for working so closely with me throughout the process. A very special thank you to Beth, who initially found my work and saw potential in it, for believing in me even in the moments I didn't believe in myself. Not only have you helped me so much creatively and given me such thorough feedback, but you have been such a support and source of encouragement.

Finally, thank you to anyone who follows WorryWellbeing for helping me create a platform to talk about mental health, for your kind comments and messages, for sharing my posts and for being part of the community that has helped me so much on my journey to recovery.

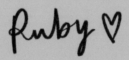

Resources

GENERAL MENTAL HEALTH RESOURCES

UK

Beder: beder.org.uk

Mental Health Foundation UK: www.mentalhealth.org.uk

Mind UK: www.mind.org.uk

Rethink Mental Illness: www.rethink.org

Samaritans: www.samaritans.org helpline 116 123

Scottish Association for Mental Health (SAMH): www.samh.org.uk

Self Care Is For Everyone: selfcareisforeveryone.com

Shout: www.giveusashout.org text 85258

Young Minds: www.youngminds.org.uk

Europe

Mental Health Europe: www.mhe-sme.org

Mental Health Ireland: www.mentalhealthireland.ie

USA

Mentalhealth.gov: www.mentalhealth.gov

Mental Health America: www.mhanational.org

National Alliance on Mental Illness (NAMI): www.nami.org

National Institute of Mental Health: www.nimh.nih.gov

Very Well Mind: www.verywellmind.com

Canada

Canadian Mental Health Association: cmha.ca

Crisis Service Canada: www.ementalhealth.ca

Australia and New Zealand

Beyond Blue: www.beyondblue.org.au

Head to Health: headtohealth.gov.au

Health Direct: www.healthdirect.gov.au

Mental Health Australia: mhaustralia.org

Mental Health Foundation of New Zealand: www.mentalhealth.org.nz

SANE Australia: www.sane.org

ANXIETY-SPECIFIC RESOURCES

UK

Anxiety UK: www.anxietyuk.org.uk

No More Panic: www.nomorepanic.co.uk

No panic: www.nopanic.org.uk

Social Anxiety: www.social-anxiety.org.uk

USA

Anxiety and Depression Association of America: www.adaa.org

Canada

Anxiety Canada: www.anxietycanada.com

Australia and New Zealand

Anxiety New Zealand Trust: www.anxiety.org.nz

Black Dog Institute: www.blackdoginstitute.org.au

SUPPORT FOR SUICIDAL THOUGHTS

UK

Campaign Against Living Miserably (CALM): www.thecalmzone.net

PAPYRUS (dedicated to the prevention of young suicide): www.papyrus-uk.org

The Samaritans: www.samaritans.org

USA

American Foundation for Suicide Prevention: afsp.org

National Suicide Prevention Lifeline: suicidepreventionlifeline.org

Canada

Canada Suicide Prevention Crisis Service: www.crisisservicescanada.ca

Australia and New Zealand

Lifeline Australia: www.lifeline.org.au

BOOKS

Chatterjee, Dr Rangan, *The Four Pillar Plan* (Penguin, 2017)

Curtis, Scarlett, *It's Not OK to Feel Blue (and Other Lies)* (Penguin, 2020)

Novogratz, Sukey, & Novogratz, Elizabeth, *Just Sit: A meditation guidebook for people who know they should but don't* (Harper Wave, 2017)

Macksey, Charlie, *The Boy the Fox and the Mole* (Ebury, 2019)

Reading, Suzy, *Self-care for Tough Times* (Aster, 2021)

Reading, Suzy, *The Self-care Revolution* (Aster, 2017)

Wax, Ruby, *How to be Human* (Penguin Life, 2018)

Weintraub, Amy, *Yoga for Depression* (Broadway Books, 2003)

ABOUT US

Welbeck Balance publishes books dedicated to changing lives. Our mission is to deliver life-enhancing books to help improve your wellbeing so that you can live your life with greater clarity and meaning, wherever you are on life's journey. Our Trigger books are specifically devoted to opening up conversations about mental health and wellbeing.

Welbeck Balance and Trigger are part of the Welbeck Publishing Group – a globally recognized independent publisher based in London. Welbeck are renowned for our innovative ideas, production values and developing long-lasting content. Our books have been translated into over 30 languages in more than 60 countries around the world.

If you love books, then join the club and sign up to our newsletter for exclusive offers, extracts, author interviews and more information.

www.welbeckpublishing.com   www.triggerhub.org

🐦 welbeckpublish   🐦 Triggercalm
📷 welbeckpublish   📷 Triggercalm
f welbeckuk   f Triggercalm

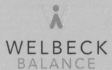

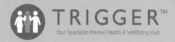